PLANT-BASED DIET

FOR BEGINNERS

Energize Your Body With Many Affordable and Delicious Recipes

Kelly Hamilton

Table of Contents

Introduction

It is only until recently that more and more people are starting to embrace the plant-based diet lifestyle. As to what exactly has drawn tens of millions of people into this lifestyle is debatable. However, there is growing evidence demonstrating that following a primarily plant-based diet lifestyle leads to better weight control and general health, free of many chronic diseases. This book will take you through the basics of this lifestyle, its benefits and why it works, as well as give ideas on how you can revamp your pantry and start whipping up delectable plant-based dishes. Whether you are new to this lifestyle or familiar with it, this book is definitely a treasure. Enjoy!

Chapter 1: The Basics of a Plant-Based Diet

What Is A Plant-Based Diet?

A lot of people are doing it; a lot of people are talking about it, but there is still a lot of confusion about what a whole food plant-based diet really means. Because we break food into its macronutrients: carbohydrates, proteins, and fats; most of us get confused about how to eat. What if we could put back together those macronutrients again so that you can free your mind of confusion and stress? Simplicity is the key here.

Whole foods are unprocessed foods that come from the earth. Now, we do eat some minimally processed foods on a whole foods plant-based diet such as whole bread, whole wheat pasta, tofu, non-dairy milk and some nuts and seed butter. All these are fine as long as they are minimally processed. So, here are the different categories:

⏥ Whole grains

⏥ Legumes (basically lentils and beans)

⏥ Fruits and vegetables

⏥ Nuts and seeds (including nut butter)

⏥ Herbs and spices

All the above-mentioned categories make up a whole foods plant-based diet. Where the fun comes in is in how you prepare them; how you season and cook them; and how you mix and match to give them great flavor and variety in your meals. There are chapters in this book dedicated to plant-based recipes which can give you an idea of what you can whip up real quick in your kitchen or those special meals you can prepare for the family. As long as you are eating foods like these on a regular basis, you can forget about carbs, protein and fat forever.

Now, some people might say, *"well, I can't eat soy"* or *"I don't like tofu"* and so on. Well, the beauty of a whole food plant based diet is that if you don't like a certain food, like in this case, soy, then you don't have to consume it. It is not a necessary component in a whole food plant-based diet. You can have brown rice instead of oats, quinoa instead of wheat; I'm sure you catch the drift now. It doesn't really matter. Just find something that suits you.

Just because you have made the decision to adopt a plant-based diet lifestyle, doesn't mean that is a healthy diet. Plant-based diets have their fair share of junk and other unhealthy eats; case and point, regular consumption of veggie pizzas and non-dairy ice cream. Staying healthy requires you to eat healthy foods – even within a plant-based diet setting.

Why You Need to Cut Back On Processed and Animal-Based Products

You've probably heard time and time again that processed food is bad for you. "Avoid preservatives; avoid processed foods"; however, no one ever really gives you any real or solid information on why you should avoid them and why they are dangerous. So let's break it down so that you can fully understand why you should avoid these culprits.

They have huge addictive properties

As humans, we really have a strong tendency to be addicted to certain foods, but the fact is that it's not entirely our fault.

Practically all of the unhealthy eats we indulge in, from time to time, activate our brains dopamine neurotransmitter. This makes the brain feel "good" but only for a short period of time. This also creates an addiction tendency; that is why someone will always find themselves going back for another candy bar – even though they don't really need it. You can avoid all this by removing that stimulus altogether.

They are loaded sugar and high fructose corn syrup

Processed and animal-based products are loaded with sugars and high fructose corn syrup which have close to zero nutritional value. More and more studies are now proving what a lot of people suspected all along; that genetically modified foods cause gut inflammation which in turn makes it harder for the body to absorb essential nutrients. The downside of your body failing to properly absorb essential nutrients, from muscle loss and brain fog to fat gain, cannot be stressed enough.

They are loaded with refined carbohydrates

Processed foods and animal-based products are loaded with refined carbs. Yes, it is a fact that your body needs carbs to provide energy to run body functions. However, refining carbs eliminates the essential nutrients; in the way that refining whole grains eliminates the whole grain component. What you are left with after refining is what's referred to as "empty" carbs. These can have a negative impact on your metabolism by spiking your blood sugar and insulin levels.

They are loaded with artificial ingredients

When your body is consuming artificial ingredients, it treats them as a foreign object. They essentially become an invader. Your body isn't used to recognizing things like sucralose or these artificial sweeteners. So, your body does what it does best. It triggers an immune response which lowers your resistance making you vulnerable to diseases. The focus and energy spent by your body in protecting your immune system could otherwise be diverted elsewhere.

What this means is that they contain components like monosodium glutamate (MSG), components of high fructose corn syrup and certain dyes that can actually carve addictive properties. They stimulate your body to get a reward out of it. MSG, for instance, is in a lot of pre-packaged pastries. What this does is that it stimulates your taste buds to enjoy the taste. It becomes psychological just by the way your brain communicates with your taste buds.

This reward-based system makes your body want more and more of it putting you at a serious risk of caloric overconsumption.

What about animal protein? Often times the term "low quality" is thrown around to refer to plant proteins since they tend to have lower amounts of essential amino acids compared to animal protein. What most people do not realize is that more essential amino acids can be quite damaging to your health. So, let's quickly explain how.

Animal Protein Lacks Fiber

In their quest to load up on more animal protein most people end up displacing the plant protein that they already had. This is bad because unlike plant protein, animal protein often lacks in fiber, antioxidants, and phytonutrients. Fiber deficiency is quite common across different communities and societies in the world. In the USA, for instance, according to the

Institute of Medicine, the average adult consumes just about 15 grams of fiber per day against the recommended 38 grams. Lack of adequate dietary fiber intake is associated with an increased risk of colon and breast cancers, as well as Crohn's disease, heart disease, and constipation.

Animal protein causes a spike in IGF-1

IGF-1 is the hormone insulin-like growth factor-1. It stimulates cell division and growth, which may sound like a good thing but it also stimulates the growth of cancer cells. Higher blood levels of IGF-1 are thus associated with increased cancer risks, malignancy, and proliferation.

Animal Protein causes an increase in Phosphorus

Animal protein contains high levels of phosphorus. Our bodies normalize the high levels of phosphorus by secreting a hormone called fibroblast growth factor 23 (FGF23). This hormone has been found to be harmful to our blood vessels, thanks to a 2013 study titled, *"Circulating Fibroblast Growth Factor 23 Is Associated with Angiographic Severity and Extent of Coronary Artery Disease"*. FGF23 has also been found to cause irregular enlargement of cardiac muscles – a risk factor for heart failure and even death in extreme cases.

Given all the issues, the "high quality" aspect of animal protein might be more appropriately described as "high risk" instead. Unlike caffeine, which you will experience withdrawal once you cut it off completely, processed foods can be cut off instantaneously. Perhaps the one thing that you'll miss is the convenience of not having to prepare every meal from scratch.

Plant-Based Diet vs. Vegan

It is quite common for people to mistake a vegan diet for a plant-based diet or vice versa. Well, even though both diets share similarities, they are not exactly the same. So let's break it down real quick.

Vegan

A vegan diet is one that contains no animal-based products. This includes meat, dairy, eggs as well as animal-derived products or ingredients such as honey. Someone who describes themselves as a vegan carries over this perspective into their everyday life. What this means is that they do not use or promote the use of clothes, shoes, accessories, shampoo, and makeups that have been made using material that comes from animals. Examples here include wool, beeswax, leather, gelatin, silk, and lanolin.

The motivation for people to lead a veganism lifestyle often stems from a desire to make a stand and fight against animal mistreatment and poor ethical treatment of animals as well as to promote animal rights.

Plant Based Diet

A whole food plant based diet in the other hand shares a similarity with veganism in the sense that it also does not promote dietary consumption of animal-based products. This includes dairy, meat, and eggs. What's more is that, unlike the vegan diet, processed foods, white flour, oils and refined sugars are not part of the diet. The idea here is to make a diet out of minimally processed to unprocessed fruits, veggies, whole grains, nuts, seeds, and legumes. So, there will be NO Oreo cookies for you.

Whole-food plant-based diet followers are often driven by the health benefits it brings. It is a diet that has very little to do with restricting calories or counting macros but mostly to do with preventing and reversing illnesses.

Getting Started on a Whole Food Plant-Based Diet

A common misconception among many people – even some of those in the health and fitness industry is that anyone who switches to a plant-based diet automatically becomes super healthy. There are tons of plant-based junk foods out there such as non-dairy ice cream and frozen veggie pizza, which can really derail your health goals if you are constantly consuming them. Committing to healthy foods is the only way that you can achieve health benefits. On the other hand, these plant-based snacks do play a role in keeping you motivated. They should be consumed in moderation, sparingly and in small bits. As you will come to see later on in this book, there is a chapter dedicated to giving ideas on plant-based snacks you can whip up at home. So, without further ado, this is how you get started on a whole food plant-based recipe.

Decide What a Plant-Based Diet Means for You

Making a decision to structure how your plant-based diet is going to look is the first step, and it is going to help you transition from your current diet outlook. This is something that is really personal and varies from one person to the other. While some people decide that they will not tolerate any animal products at all, some make do with tiny bits of dairy or meat occasionally. It is really up to you to decide what and how you want your plant-based diet to look like. The most important thing is that whole plant-based foods have to make a great majority of your diet.

Understand What You Are Eating

All right, now that you've gotten the decision part down, your next task is going to involve a lot of analysis on your part. What do we mean by this? Well, if this is your first time trying out the plant-based diet, you may be surprised by the number of foods, especially packaged foods, which contain animal products. You will find yourself nurturing the habit of reading labels while you are shopping. Turns out, lots of pre-packaged foods have animal products in them, so if you want to stick only to plant products for your new diet, you'll need to keep a keen eye on ingredient labels. Perhaps you decided to allow some amount of animal products in your diet; well, you are still going to have to watch out for foods loaded with fats, sugars, sodium, preservatives and other things that could potentially impact your healthy diet.

Find Revamped Versions of Your Favorite Recipes

I'm sure you have a number of favorite dishes that are not necessarily plant-based. For most people, leaving all that behind is usually the hardest part. However, there is still a way you could meet halfway. Take some time to ponder what you like about those non-plant based meals. Think along the lines of flavor, texture, versatility and so on; and look for swaps in the whole food plant-based diet that can fulfill what you will be missing. Just to give you some insight into what I mean, here are a couple of examples:

- Crumbled or blended tofu would make for a decent filling in both sweet and savory dishes just like ricotta cheese would in lasagna.
- Lentils go particularly well with saucy dishes that are typically associated with meatloaf and Bolognese.

As you read on, you will come across a chapter dedicated to an assortment of delectable main course recipes that are purely plant-based. All in all, when this is executed right, you will not even miss your non-plant based favorite meals.

Build a Support Network

Building any new habit is tough, but it doesn't have to be. Find yourself some friends, or even relatives, who are willing to lead this lifestyle with you. This will help you stay focused and motivated while also providing emotional support and some form of accountability. You can do fun stuff like trying out and sharing new recipes with these friends or even hitting up restaurants that offer a variety of plant-based options. You can even go a step further and look up local plant-based groups on social media to help you expand your knowledge and support network.

Chapter 2: What You Stand to Gain from a Plant-Based Diet

The Benefits of Going Plant-Based

More and more people are becoming aware of the ability of a whole food plant based diet to help alleviate and even cure many chronic diseases such as heart disease, type 2 diabetes, arthritis, cancers, autoimmune disease, kidney stones, inflammatory bowel diseases and many more. Not to mention, a plant-based diet is more economical – especially when you buy local organic produce that is in season. So let's check out some of the benefits of going plant-based.

- **It Lowers Blood Pressure**

  Plant-based foods tend to have a higher amount of potassium whose benefits, notably include: reducing blood pressure and alleviating stress and anxiety. Some foods rich in potassium include legumes, nuts, seeds, whole grains, and fruits. Meat, on the other hand, contains very little to no potassium.

- **It Lowers Cholesterol**

  Plants contain NO cholesterol – even the saturated sources like cacao and coconut. Leading a plant-based lifestyle will, therefore, help you lower the levels of cholesterol in your body leading to reduced risks of heart disease.

- **Checks Your Blood Sugar Levels**

  Plant-based foods tend to have a lot of fiber. This helps slow down the absorption of sugars into the bloodstream as well as keep you feeling full for longer periods of time. It also helps balance out your blood cortisol levels thereby reducing stress.

- **It Helps Prevent and Fight Off Chronic Diseases**

  In societies where a majority of people lead a plant-based lifestyle the rates of chronic diseases such as cancer, obesity, and diabetes are usually very low. This diet has also been proven to lengthen the lives of those already suffering from these chronic diseases.

- **It Is Good for Weight Loss**

  Consuming whole plant-based foods make it easier to cut off excess weight and maintain a healthier weight without having to involve calorie restrictions. This is because Weight loss naturally occurs when you consume more fiber, vitamins, and minerals than you do animal fats and proteins.

What Some Influential People Think of a Plant-Based Lifestyle

Whether we like to admit it or not, celebrities do have a lot of fame and power, which can either be used to promote good or promote evil. Going plant-based can be quite a daunting experience as it often comes with a health and lifestyle overhaul, however, nowadays it's become an increasingly popular diet – and a host of stars have made the change. We have already explored some of the numerous benefits of going plant-based. Some celebrities are passively plant-based diet followers; this means that they are not celebrities because of their diet views, but became a celebrity as a result of something else like their music or roles in the film industry. Others are active plant-based diet followers whose claim to fame is adding something of value to the conversation of a plant-based diet and lifestyle. Let's look at some celebrities who subscribe to this lifestyle and what they have to say.

Liam Hemsworth who's an acclaimed actor known for many film roles among which include, The Hunger Games once said this to Men's Fitness Magazine about the plant-based diet, *"I feel nothing but positive, mentally and physically. I love it. I feel like it also has a kind of a domino effect on the rest of my life"*.

Jennifer Lopez, a well-known and talented singer and actress, after the giving birth to her twins, had this to say about plant-based diet: *"It is a real change, but more than that I feel better and people are like 'Your energy's better'."*

Jenna Dewan Tatum made the jump from vegetarian to vegan a couple of years ago. She says, *"After going vegan, I felt so much better. My skin cleared up, I had a ton more energy and I just felt clearer in the head"*.

Ariana Grande is yet another plant-based diet follower who shares a trick she employs when dining out. She says, *"It is tricky dining out, but I just stick to what I know – veggies, fruit and salad - then when I get home I'll have something else."*

Taj McWilliams-Franklin, a professional basketball player, was quoted in a 2008 interview about why she decided to go plant-based saying, *"I just wanted to make sure I had a healthy body because I wanted to continue playing for a longer period than most of my peers."*

What to Look Out For When Adopting this Lifestyle

For most people looking to go plant-based, protein is always a major concern. There is this notion that's perpetuated by the mainstream media backed by big meat producers that protein is only found in meat. Well, that's just not true. Traditional staples such as nuts, beans, oats and brown rice come with a lot of protein.

Often times, nutrients like calcium are also marketed as coming from only animal-based sources. The truth is that foods like kale, broccoli, and almonds contain lots of calcium. Ask yourself this, if calcium comes from meat, then where did the animal get it from? It's definitely from the greens they eat.

The major concern for most plant-based diet followers is usually vitamin B12. B12, for everyone, is usually found in fortified products, especially cereals and plant-based milk. However, those shouldn't be relied on to get enough of this important vitamin. The best option is to take a liquid or sublingual vitamin B12 supplement simply; just to make sure that there are no issues.

You can adopt a healthy plant-based lifestyle by basing your diet around cooked and raw foods filled with leafy and colorful veggies. These will provide your body with the minerals, vitamins, and antioxidants it needs.

Chapter 3: Planning and Stocking Your Pantry

A Quick word on Pantry Planning

As you transition into a whole-food, plant-based lifestyle, you don't have to worry about stocking. Your local farmer's market or grocery store should provide you with everything you need. Consider getting sets of transparent jars which you will use to store your food. This will make for a presentable look in your pantry. Typically, you will have some shelves dedicated to storage of grains, nuts, beans, spices, herbs and so on.

Stock Your Pantry: Food Guide for a Plant-Based Diet

Foods to Stock

Non-Starchy Vegetables

- Leafy greens (Kale, Spinach, Butter Lettuce etc.)

- Broccoli

- Zucchini

- Eggplant

- Tomatoes

Starchy Vegetables

- All kinds of potatoes

- Whole corn

- Legumes (all beans and lentils)

- Root vegetables

- Quinoa

Fruits

- All whole fruits (avoid dried and juiced fruits)

Whole Grains

- 100% whole wheat, brown rice, and oats

Beverages

- Water

- Green tea

- Unsweetened plant-based milk

- Decaffeinated coffee and tea

Spices

- All spices

Omega 3 Sources

- Ground flax seed
- Chia seeds

Nuts

- Peanuts
- Almonds
- Cashews
- Walnuts

Foods to Consume Sparingly

- Avocadoes
- Coconuts
- Sesame seeds
- Sunflower seeds

- Pumpkin seeds

- Dried fruit

- Added sweeteners (maple syrup, fruit juice concentrate, and natural sugars)

- Caffeinated tea and coffee

- Alcoholic beverages

- Refined soy protein and wheat protein

Foods to Avoid

Meat

- Fish

- Poultry

- Seafood

- Red meat

- Processed meat

Dairy

- Yogurt

- Milk

- Cheese

- Cream

- Half and half

- Buttermilk

Added Fats

- Liquid oils

- Coconut oil

- Margarine

- Butter

Beverages

- Soda

- Fruit juice

- Sports drinks

- Energy drinks

- Blended coffee and tea drinks

Refined Flours

- All wheat flours that are not 100% whole wheat

Vegan Replacement Foods

- Vegan "cheese" or vegan "meats" containing any oil

Miscellaneous

- Eggs

- Candy bars

- Pastries

- Cookies

- Cakes

- Energy bars

A Quick Word on Labels

When shopping to restock your pantry, always keep in mind that the goal is not to eat a lot of foods that require packaging or labels. However, it is normal to have that packaged food item on your list occasionally. When this does happen, these tips will help you stay vigilant and ensure a healthy shopping experience.

Do Not Believe Company Claims

Terms like 'low in fat' or '50% less sodium' are very popular on packaged foods. They don't really mean anything. What you should instead be focusing on is the ingredient list and the nutrition label. Just because a bag of potato chips has been labeled as having 40% less sodium doesn't mean that it is healthy. It could very well be still high in sodium or come with a host of other unwanted ingredients. The same goes for products labeled as "low-fat."

Make a Habit of Checking the Ingredient List

As a general rule, the fewer ingredients there are, the healthier the food is. Such foods often have very few to no additives and preservatives which is good for your health. When you see the ingredients list containing a lot of words ending in "-ose," this is often an indicator that the food contains a lot of sugar. Also, check if there are any animal products on the ingredient list.

Chapter 4: Breakfast and Brunch Recipes

Maple Granola with Banana Whipped Topping

Ingredients

- 2 cups of rolled oats

- ¼ cup of raw sunflower seeds

- ¼ cup of raw pumpkin seeds

- ¼ cup of raw unsweetened shredded dried coconut

- ¼ cup chopped walnuts

- ¼ cup raw or toasted wheat germ

- 1 teaspoon ground cinnamon

- ½ cup maple syrup

- ¾ cup raisins

- Banana Whipped Topping, optional

For Banana Whipped Topping

- 8 ounces soft or firm regular tofu, drained (sprouted variety is preferred)

- 1 ripe banana

- 2 tablespoons maple syrup, plus more as needed

Instructions

i. Line a baking sheet with parchment paper and preheat your oven to 330 degrees F.

ii. Combine oats, pumpkin seeds, walnuts, sunflower seeds, cinnamon and wheat germ in a bowl along with maple syrup.

iii. Now in your baking sheet, spread the mixture evenly and bake for about 20 minutes.

iv. Stir in raisins and bake for another 5 minutes until the oats are golden.

v. Transfer to another baking sheet or tray and let it cool. You can serve it with banana toppings.

For Topping

Combine topping ingredients in a blender until smooth. Add maple syrup as desired.

Chickpea Flour Scramble

Ingredients

Chickpea flour batter:

- ½ cup of chickpea flour or use ½ cup + 1 or 2 tablespoons of more gram flour

- ½ cup of water

- 1 tablespoon of nutritional yeast

- 1 tablespoon of flaxseed meal

- ½ teaspoon of baking powder

- ¼ teaspoon of salt

- ¼ teaspoon of turmeric

- ¼ teaspoon or less paprika

- 1/8 teaspoon of Indian Sulphur black salt for the eggy flavor

- Generous dash of black pepper

For Veggies:

- 1 teaspoon of oil divided

- 1 clove of garlic

- ¼ cup chopped onions

- 2 tablespoons each of asparagus green bell pepper, zucchini or other veggies.

- ½ green chili, chopped

- 2 tablespoons of chopped red bell pepper or tomato

- Cilantro and black pepper for garnish

Instructions

i. Blend all the ingredients under chickpea flour batter and keep aside. You can also use lentil batter from my lentil frittata.

ii. Heat ½ teaspoon of oil in a skillet over medium heat. Add onion and garlic and cook for about 3 minutes until translucent.

iii. Add veggies, chili and cook for another 2 mins, then add spices and greens.

iv. Cover the veggies with the chickpea flour batter and continue cooking while adding olive oil.

v. Since the mixture tends to get doughy, be sure to scrap the bottom. Cook until the edges dry out. This should take about 5 minutes.

vi. Turn off the stove and break the food into smaller chunks then season with salt and pepper. You can garnish with cilantro if you like. Serve with toast or tacos.

Peanut Butter and Jam Porridge

Ingredients

Peanut butter granola

- ½ cup of rolled oats or an assortment of cereals/nuts/seeds in your pantry

- 1 tablespoon peanut butter

- 1 teaspoon of rice malt syrup

Raspberry chia jam

- ¼ cup raspberries

- 1 tablespoon chia seeds

Porridge

- ⅔ Cup of rolled oats

- 1½ cup of coconut milk

- 2 tablespoon of peanut butter (optional)

- 1 banana, mashed (optional)

Other toppings

- 2 tablespoon of peanut butter

- Whatever you desire! (Such as cacao nibs, coconut syrup, coconut and frozen berries)

Instructions

i. Preheat oven to 360°F.

ii. Combine granola ingredients in a baking sheet and bake for about 10 minutes (or until golden brown)

iii. Mash raspberries and mix in chia seeds then set it aside.

iv. Combine all porridge ingredients in a saucepan and bring to boil. Stir occasionally to maintain its smoothness.

v. Separate the porridge into 2 bowls and add granola, chia seeds, and peanut butter as desired.

Banana Almond Granola

- 8 cups rolled oats

- 2 cups pitted and chopped dates

- 2 ripe bananas, peeled and chopped

- 1 teaspoon almond extract

- 1 teaspoon salt

- 1 cup slivered almonds, toasted (optional)

Instructions

i. Preheat the oven to 275°F.

ii. Line a baking sheet with parchment paper.

iii. Cook dates covered with water in a saucepan over medium heat for about 10 minutes. Make sure the dates do not stick on the pan.

iv. Take the mixture off heat and in a blender, combine it with almond extract, bananas and salt until creamy.

v. Add oats to the date mixture and spread out on the baking sheet. Bake for about 45 minutes – occasionally stirring.

vi. Remove from oven and let it cool. Enjoy.

Polenta with Pears and Cranberries

- ¼ cup of brown rice syrup

- 2 pears, peeled, cored, and diced

- 1 cup of fresh or dried cranberries

- 1 teaspoon ground cinnamon

- 1 batch Basic Polenta, kept warm

i. In a medium saucepan, combine the brown rice syrup, cranberries, pears and cinnamon. Cook until the pears are tender.

ii. Divide as desired and top with pear compote.

Fruit and Nut Oatmeal

- ¾ cup of rolled oats

- ¼ teaspoon ground cinnamon

- Pinch of sea salt

- ¼ cup fresh berries (optional)

- ½ ripe banana, sliced (optional)

- 2 tablespoons of chopped nuts, such as walnuts, pecans, or cashews (optional)

- 2 tablespoons of dried fruit, such as raisins, cranberries, chopped apples, chopped

- Apricots (optional)

- Maple syrup (optional)

i. Cook oats in water in a saucepan until it starts boiling. Reduce the heat and let it simmer for about 5 minutes.

ii. Add cinnamon and salt – stirring. Top with berries and fruits and serve while hot.

Red Pesto and Kale Porridge

Ingredients

- ½ cup of oats

- ½ cup of couscous

- 2 cups of veggie stock (or water)

- 1 teaspoon of dried oregano

- 1 teaspoon of dried basil

- 1 cup of chopped kale

- 1 cup of sliced cherry tomatoes

- 1 scallion

- 1 teaspoon of tahini

- 1 tablespoon of pesto of your choice

- 2 tablespoons of nutritional yeast

- 1 tablespoon of pumpkin seed

- 1 tablespoon of hemp seed

- Salt and pepper to taste

Instructions

i.   Cook oats, couscous, vegetable stock, oregano, basil, salt and pepper in a small pot on medium heat for about 5 minutes stirring occasionally.

ii. Once it becomes creamy, add scallions, chopped kale, and tomatoes. Stir in pesto, yeast, and tahini.

iii. Top with some cherry tomatoes hemp seeds and pumpkin and serve it warm.

Spicy Tofu Scramble

Ingredients

- 350g of firm tofu

- 2 small spring onions, sliced

- 1 large garlic clove, finely chopped

- 10 cherry tomatoes, halved

- ½ fresh red chili, sliced

- 1 avocado, sliced

- 1 teaspoon of ground turmeric

- 2 teaspoon of ground black salt

- Salt & pepper to taste

- 1 to 2 tablespoons of olive oil

- 8 slices of gluten-free bread, toasted

Instructions

i. Sauté garlic in olive oil in a pan.

ii. Add in tomatoes and cook until they're soft then remove the mixture from the pan.

iii. Under a grill, toast bread slices. Sauté some onions and chili seeds on low-medium heat until they soften and add tofu.

iv. Sprinkle with turmeric and black salt and stir it for a couple of minutes. Finally, add tomatoes and garlic back to the pan to warm up.

v. Add the tofu scramble onto the toasted bread slices and decorate with avocado. Season as desired. Enjoy!

Green Chia Pudding

- 1 Medjool date with pit removed

- 1 cup non-dairy milk organic soy, almond, or coconut

- 1 handful fresh spinach

- 3 tablespoons of chia seeds

- Fruit for topping banana, kiwi, mango or berries

i. Combine the dates, milk, and spinach in a blender until smooth then add it to chia seeds in a medium bowl.

ii. Store in the refrigerator for up to overnight.

iii. Top with fruit before serving.

Turmeric Steel Cut Oats

Ingredients

- ¼ teaspoon of olive oil

- ½ cup of steel cut oats use certified gluten-free if needed

- 1½ cup of water 2 cups for a thinner consistency

- 1 cup of non-dairy milk

- 1/3 teaspoon of turmeric

- ½ teaspoon of cinnamon

- ¼ teaspoon of cardamom

- Salt to taste

- 2 tablespoons or more, of maple or other sweetener of your choice

Instructions

i.   Toast oats in oil in a saucepan for a couple of minutes.

ii. Add water and milk and bring it to a boil before letting it simmer.

iii. Mix in the spices, salt, and maple and cook for about 8 minutes or until the oats

     are cooked to preference.

iv. Taste and adjust sweet, and flavors as desired then let it cool to thicken. You can serve warm or chilled.

v.   Garnish with strawberries, dried fruit or chia seeds.

Chapter 5: Main Course Recipes

Mashed Cauliflower and Green Bean Casserole

Ingredients

- ¾ cup of coconut milk

- ½ cup of nutritional yeast

- 1 cauliflower

- Salt and pepper to taste

- 14 ounces of green beans, trimmed

- 1 onion, diced

Instructions

i.   In a skillet, cook cauliflower florets in vegetable broth and some olive oil.

ii. Add in onions and beans and cook for a little longer. Transfer the mixture into a blender and add coconut milk, nutritional yeast, salt and pepper and blend until smooth.

iii. In a baking sheet, assemble green bean mix, mashed cauliflower, and toppings and bake for 15 to 20 minutes at 400 degrees F. Enjoy.

Zucchini Noodles with Portobello Bolognese

Ingredients

- 3 tablespoons extra virgin olive oil, divided

- 6 Portobello mushroom caps, stems, and gills removed and finely chopped

- ½ cup of minced carrot

- ½ cup of minced celery

- ½ cup of minced yellow onion

- 3 large garlic cloves, minced

- Kosher salt

- Fresh ground pepper

- 1 tablespoon of tomato paste

- A 28-ounce can crushed tomatoes (I strongly recommend San Marzano)

- 2 teaspoons of dried oregano

- ¼ teaspoon of crushed red pepper (optional)

- ½ cup fresh basil leaves, finely chopped (plus extra for serving)

- 4 medium zucchini

Instructions

i.   Sauté garlic, mushrooms, celery, and carrots in olive oil in a pan. Season with salt and pepper as desired. Continue cooking until vegetables are soft.

ii.   Stir in some tomato paste and cook for a couple of minutes before adding crushed tomatoes, oregano, red pepper, and basil.

iii.   Let it simmer for 10 to 15 minutes until the sauce thickens.

iv.   As the sauce simmers, use an appropriate blade to make spiral zucchini.

v.   Sauté the zucchini noodles in a separate saucepan for a couple of minutes and season as desired.

vi.   Top with a generous amount of Bolognese and garnish with freshly chopped basil and serve immediately.

Burrito Bowl

- Baked tortilla chips

- 2 to 4 cups cooked grains

- 2 to 4 cups cooked beans

- 2 to 4 cups chopped romaine lettuce or steamed kale

- 2 to 4 chopped tomatoes

- 1 to 2 chopped green onions

- 1 to 2 cups corn kernels

- 1 avocado, chopped

- Fresh salsa

i. Break some tortilla chips and place in a bowl.

ii. Add some cooked grains and beans.

iii. Layer on tomatoes, lettuce, corn, onions, avocado and then top with salsa.

Thai Noodles

Ingredients

- 8 ounces brown rice noodles or other whole-grain noodles

- 3 tablespoons of low-sodium soy sauce, or to taste

- 2 tablespoons of brown rice syrup or maple syrup

- 2 tablespoons of fresh lime juice (from 1 to 2 limes)

- 4 garlic cloves, minced

- 3 cups of frozen Asian-style vegetables

- 1 cup of mung bean sprouts

- 2 green onions, white and light green parts chopped

- 3 tablespoons of chopped, roasted, unsalted peanuts

- ¼ cup of chopped fresh cilantro

- 1 lime, cut into wedges

Instructions

i. Follow instructions for cooking noodles.

ii. Combine soy sauce, garlic, brown rice syrup, lime juice and cup water and bring to a boil. Stir in the veggies and cook for about 5 minutes or until crisp-tender.

iii. Add the cooked noodles and mung bean sprouts and toss to coat then let it cook for a couple more minutes.

iv. Garnish with cilantro, green onions, lime wedges and chopped peanuts.

Mediterranean Vegetable Spaghetti

- 10 ounces brown rice spaghetti

- 1 red bell pepper, cubed small

- 1 yellow bell pepper, cubed small

- 2 plum tomatoes, sliced into eighths (discard the seeds)

- Salt

- ½ jalapeño (optional)

- 2 tablespoons of dried herbs de Provence

- 2 tablespoons of tomato purée

- 2 tablespoons apple cider vinegar or juice of 1 lime

- 12 cherry tomatoes, quartered

- 1 zucchini, halved then sliced into thin half-rounds

- 1 bunch spinach, chopped

- Handful of black olives

i. Cook pasta, drain and set aside.

ii. Sauté peppers, tomatoes, jalapeno, and herbs in a saucepan. Add water and let it simmer.

iii. Add tomato puree and vinegar or lime juice and let it cook together for a few minutes until it becomes saucy.

iv. Add cherry tomatoes, zucchini slices, and spinach. Mix well and cook for about 5 to 7 minutes.

v. Add olives and sauce to the pasts along with some herbs. Enjoy

Mexican Lentil Soup

- 2 tablespoons extra virgin olive oil

- 1 yellow onion, diced

- 2 carrots, peeled and diced

- 2 celery stalks, diced

- 1 red bell pepper, diced

- 3 cloves garlic, minced

- 1 tablespoon cumin

- ¼ teaspoon smoked paprika

- 1 teaspoon oregano

- 2 cups diced tomatoes and the juices

- 4 ounces diced green chilies

- 2 cups green lentils, rinsed and picked over

- 8 cups vegetable broth

- ½ teaspoon salt

- A dash (or more) of hot sauce, plus more for serving

- Fresh cilantro, for garnish

- 1 avocado, peeled, pitted, and diced, or garnish

Instructions

i. Sauté onions, celery, bell pepper and carrots in a pan for about 5 minutes then add garlic, cumin, paprika, and oregano and let it cook for another minute.

ii. Add in tomatoes, chilies, lentils, broth, and salt to taste and bring to a simmer until lentils are tender.

iii. Season with salt and pepper as necessary

iv. Serve it garnished with fresh cilantro, avocado, and a few dashes of hot sauce.

Walnut Meat Tacos

Ingredients

Walnut Tacos:

- 1½ cups de-shelled walnuts

- 1 teaspoon of garlic powder

- ½ teaspoon of cumin

- ½ teaspoon of chili powder

- A tablespoon of tamari

- 6 Taco shells (organic & gluten-free)

Toppings:

- 1 cup carrots chopped

- 1 cup red cabbage chopped

- ¼ cup of onion, chopped

- Cilantro chopped

Lime Cashew Sour Cream:

- 1 Cup cashews soaked overnight (or soaked at least 10 mins in boiling water)

- ½ cup of water (and more if needed)

- 2 tablespoons of lime juice

- A tablespoon of apple cider vinegar

- Pinch of salt to taste

Instructions

i. Blend walnuts in a food processor until it looks "meaty."

ii. Add walnuts to a food processor and process until mixture is kind of "meaty."

iii. Put mixture in a bowl and add seasonings and mix. Add the remaining ingredients and stir well.

iv. Fill taco shells with the mixture and top as desired.

v. Combine all ingredients of the lime cashew sour cream in a blender until smooth.

vi. Top tacos with sour cream and enjoy!

Pineapple Papaya Fried Rice

Ingredients

- 3 cups of organic brown rice, cooked and chilled

- 1 large papaya, peeled and cubed

- A can of 100% pineapple chunks only, drain the juice

- ½ cup of garden peas (organic and local if possible)

- 1 cup of mixed bell peppers (green and sweet red)

- 1 medium sized onion, diced

- 3 small scallion, chopped

- 2 tsp of Coconut Aminos

- 3 garlic cloves, minced,

- 1 tsp of turmeric

- 1 tsp of fresh ginger, minced

- ½ teaspoon of Himalayan pink salt

- 1½ teaspoon of sesame seed oil

- ½ teaspoon of white pepper

- 2 tablespoons of coconut oil

- 1 teaspoon of thyme

Instructions

i. Melt coconut oil in a large frying pan and add turmeric, onion, scallion, garlic, and ginger.

ii. Sauté until the onions are soft then add bell peppers and garden peas. Stir occasionally until the veggies are soft in texture.

iii. Once this is achieved, add papaya, pineapple and cold rice in the frying pan and stir until the mixture takes turns yellow.

iv. Drizzle the coconut aminos and sesame oil into the frying pan and flip once or twice.

v. Season with thyme, white pepper, and salt and stir thoroughly to deepen the flavor. Serve accordingly.

Garlic Hash Brown with Kale

Ingredients

- 2 Yukon Gold potatoes, shredded

- ¼ teaspoon salt

- ½ teaspoon of freshly ground black pepper

- 6 cloves garlic, minced

- 2 to 3 large kale leaves, shredded

- Pinch of salt

NOTE: You can substitute Yukon Gold potatoes with shredded sweet potatoes

Instructions

i. Preheat your oven to 375° F.

ii. Season shredded potatoes with salt and pepper and spread them on a baking sheet lined with a silicone baking mat and bake for 10 minutes.

iii. Remove it from the oven and toss with minced garlic. Return them to the oven and bake for a couple more minutes.

iv. In a large pan, over medium heat, sauté shredded kale with some water until it is soft and set aside to cool. Make sure not to add more water when it evaporates.

v. Squeeze the kale to get rid of excess water, and then toss it a bit to separate the cooked shreds.

vi. Plate the crisped potatoes, top it with the kale, and serve.

Cauliflower and Tomato Coconut Curry

Ingredients

- 1 yellow onion

- 4 cups of sweet potato, chopped

- 1 head cauliflower, chopped

- 2 tablespoons of olive oil

- 1 teaspoon kosher salt, divided

- 2 tablespoons curry powder

- 1 tablespoon garam masala

- 1 teaspoon of cumin

- ¼ teaspoon of cayenne

- 23-ounce jar of diced San Marzano plum tomatoes

- A 15-ounce can of coconut milk

- A 15-ounce can of chickpeas

- 4 cups of spinach leaves

- Cilantro, for garnish

- Brown rice, for serving

Instructions

   i.   Cook brown rice as instructed.

  ii.   Dice the onion and chop the sweet potato into bite-sized chunks (do not peel). Chop the cauliflower into florets as well.

 iii. Sauté onions in olive oil then add the sweet potato and continue cooking for 2 to 3 minutes.

 iv. Add in cauliflower and salt to taste continue cooking for a few more minutes. Now, stir in curry powder, garam masala, cumin, cayenne, tomatoes and coconut milk.

  v.   Bring to a boil, and then let it simmer for about 8 to 10 minutes until the cauliflower and sweet potato are tender.

 vi. Add in chickpeas and spinach and stir well before seasoning with salt as desired.

vii. Garnish with chopped cilantro, and serve with brown rice.

Chapter 6: Dessert and Treats Recipes

Cream Decorated Truffles

Ingredients

For the truffles:

- 2 tablespoons of organic raw cacao

- ½ cup of organic raw zucchini

- ½ cup of rolled oats

- ¼ cup Medjool dates or raisins

For the cream:

- ½ cup cashews

- ½ teaspoons of alcohol-free vanilla extract

- 2 Medjool dates, pitted

For decorating:

- 1 tablespoon filtered water

- ½ tsp. organic raw cacao

Instructions

i.   Combine truffle ingredients in a blender until fully-fused.

ii. Using wet hands form the mixture into small balls and set aside.

iii. Combine cream ingredients in a blender until smooth then spread it over some of the truffles.

iv. Add two small pea size quantities of cream for the mummies' eyeballs for the remaining truffles.

v. Mix water and cacao in a small bowl and use a toothpick to make drops of the mixture onto the truffles. Enjoy.

Raw Apple Tart

Ingredients

- 3 organic apples (of your choice), grated

- A cup of dried cranberries

- A cup of old-fashioned rolled oats

- 2 tablespoons of raw almond butter

- 1 cup of unsweetened coconut flakes

Instructions

i. Combine apples, cranberries, oats, and almond butter in a dish.

ii. Top with the coconut flakes, cover, and refrigerate for 2 hours.

Raw Orange Chocolate Pudding

Ingredients

- 1 vanilla bean, seeds scraped out (or 1 ½ tsp pure vanilla extract)

- A cup of peeled, pitted, and roughly chopped ripe avocado

- 1 cup pitted dates

- 1/3 cup raw or regular cocoa powder

- 1 teaspoon of orange zest

- ½ cup of freshly squeezed orange juice

- 1/8 teaspoon of sea salt

Instructions

i. Combine all ingredients in a food processor and puree until smooth.

ii. You can thin the puree by adding more orange juice, or a splash of nut milk or water.

iii. Serve or store in the refrigerator.

iii.

Mango Chia Seed Pudding

- 2 cups of coconut milk

- ½ cup of chia seeds

- 1 teaspoon of vanilla (powder or extract)

- ¼ teaspoon of cardamom

- 1 medium sized mango

- 3 tablespoons of coconut nectar or 2 tablespoons of date paste

i. Mix chia seeds with coconut milk, coconut nectar, vanilla, and cardamom in a bowl and refrigerate up to overnight.

ii. Slice the mango up into pieces and puree in a blender.

iii. Serve accordingly – mix together or serve in layers and enjoy!

Chewy Lemon and Oatmeal Cookies

Ingredients

- 10 dates, pitted

- A cup of unsweetened applesauce

- 1½ teaspoons of apple cider vinegar

- A cup of rolled oats

- A cup of oat flour

- ½ cup quick-cooking oats

- ¾ cup roughly chopped walnuts

- 2 tablespoons of grated lemon zest (from about 2 lemons)

- 2 teaspoons of natural cocoa powder

- 1 teaspoon of vanilla powder

- ½ teaspoon of baking soda

- Pinch of sea salt to taste

Instructions

i. Preheat the oven to 275°F and line 2 baking sheets with parchment paper.

ii. Soak the dates in hot water for about 20 minutes then blend them with applesauce and vinegar.

iii. Stir together the rolled oats, oat flour, quick-cooking oats, walnuts, lemon zest, cocoa powder, vanilla powder, baking soda, and salt in a large bowl.

iv. Mix in the dates and applesauce paste and make sure that the mixture is relatively dry.

v. Scoop a portion, roll it into a ball, pat it flat and place onto a baking sheet. Repeat this until you use up all the mixture.

vi. Bake for about 40 minutes until the tops of the cookies appear crispy and browned.

vii. Let them cool on a wire rack. Enjoy.

vii.

Chocolate Buckwheat Granola Bars

- 2 bananas

- ¼ cup of peanut butter (or almond butter)

- 1 tablespoon of cocoa powder

- 1 teaspoon of all-natural vanilla extract (I used my homemade one)

- 3 tablespoons of date syrup or maple syrup

- 1⅓ cup of buckwheat groats

- ⅓ - ½ cup of dark chocolate chunks (sweetened with healthy sweeteners if you
  can find it or you can use unsweetened and increase the date syrup by 1
  tablespoon)

i. Preheat the oven to 360 degrees F (180 degrees Celsius).

ii. Combine and mash the bananas with peanut butter, cocoa powder, vanilla extract
and date syrup in a bowl.

iii. Add chocolate and buckwheat groats and pour into a brownie pan.

iv. Bake for about 20 minutes until the granola bars firm up then set it aside to cool.

Enjoy.

Cauliflower Chocolate Pudding

- 3 cups of cauliflower florets

- 2 cups of non-dairy milk (e.g. almond milk)

- 1/3 cup of cacao powder

- 10 pitted Medjool dates

- ½ teaspoon of vanilla bean powder (or a teaspoon of vanilla extract)

Instructions

i.   Steam the cauliflower until they become tender.

ii. Combine all ingredients in a blender until smooth and creamy.

iii. You can consume immediately or store in the fridge.

Spicy Vegan Black Bean Brownies

Ingredients

- 2 tablespoons of ground flax seed plus 6 tablespoons of water, mixed well

- 1 cup (132 g) oat flour

- 1¼ cup (141 g) cacao or unsweetened cocoa powder

- 1 teaspoon of baking powder

- 1 teaspoon of finely ground sea salt

- 2 teaspoons (5 g) of ground cinnamon

- ½ teaspoon cayenne powder (optional)

- 30 ounces (878 g) of cooked black beans, drained and rinsed well

- 1 cup (240 ml) of pure maple syrup

- 2 teaspoon (10 ml) of pure vanilla extract

- ¼ (60 ml) cup water, add more by the teaspoon if needed.

Instructions

i.   Preheat the oven to 350°F (176°C) and grease a pan to make the flax eggs and let

     sit.

ii. Add the oats, cocoa powder, baking powder, salt, cinnamon, and cayenne pepper to the food processor and grind the oats into flour.

iii. Once this has been done, add in the beans, flax eggs, maple syrup, vanilla, and water and process until the batter is smooth and creamy. Use water to thin the mixture as desired.

iv. Bake for half an hour and let it cool on a rack.

Chocolate Peanut Butter High Protein Sundae

Ingredients

- 1 banana, sliced and frozen

- ½ cup of frozen cooked lentils

- ¼ cup of almond milk, or non-dairy milk of your choice

- A tablespoon peanut butter

- A tablespoon unsweetened cocoa powder

- 2 tablespoons of shelled, salted peanuts

- 2 teaspoons of cacao nibs

Instructions

i. Mix frozen banana slices and lentils with almond milk, peanut butter, and cocoa powder in a blender periodically scraping the sides.

ii. Serve in a bowl and top with peanuts and cacao nibs. Enjoy.

ii.

Berry Basil Popsicles

Ingredients

- 1½ cup of sliced strawberries

- 1 cup of mixed berries (I used raspberry, red currant, and blueberry)

- 10 to 20 fresh basil leaves

- A tablespoon of lemon juice

- 1 to 3 tablespoons of maple syrup (optional)

Instructions

i. Combine all ingredients in a blender until smooth.

ii. Pour the mixture into Popsicle molds and insert Popsicle sticks. Freeze overnight.

   Enjoy!

Chapter 7: Drinks and Smoothies Recipes

Red Velvet Cake Smoothie

Ingredients

- 2 ripe bananas, peeled

- ½ medium beet, scrubbed and roughly chopped

- ½ cup of walnut pieces

- 4 to 6 pitted dates, depending on how sweet you want it

- 1 cup fresh packed spinach

- ¼ cup of unsweetened cocoa powder

- 1 teaspoon of pure vanilla extract

- 1½ cups of non-dairy milk such as almond, rice, or coconut

- 2 cups of ice

Optional Garnish:

- Finely chopped dark chocolate

- Finely chopped walnuts

- Coconut flakes

Instructions

i.   Combine all ingredients in a blender until a smoothie consistency is achieved.

ii. Garnish as desired and serve!

Berry Soft Serve

- A large banana

- ¾ cup of frozen mixed berries

- ½ cup of nondairy milk

i. The previous night: peel banana, break into chunks, and freeze

ii. Combine frozen banana, berries, and milk in a blender and blend until creamy and thick. Add a splash of milk to thin.

iii. Serve with some vegan brownies!

Quinoa, Berry and Coconut Smoothie

Ingredients

- A cup of almond or coconut milk

- A cup of raspberries

- 1 Medjool date

- ½ cup of cooked quinoa

- 2 tablespoons of dried goji berries

- 2 tablespoons of shredded coconut

Instructions

i. Remove the pit and put the date into your blender jar. Add in the rest of the ingredients

ii. Blend for until smooth. Refrigerate or drink right away.

Blueberry Avocado Chia Smoothie

Ingredients

- A cup of blueberries

- A cup of almond coconut milk

- 1 Medjool date

- ½ of a ripe avocado

- A tablespoon of chia or flax

- ¼ teaspoon of vanilla powder

Instructions

i. Put one half of a skinned avocado in a blender jar and add the fresh or frozen blueberries, pitted date and the remaining ingredients then blend until smooth.

ii. Refrigerate or drink right away.

Strawberry Kale Smoothie

- A cup of strawberries

- ½ a banana

- A cup of kale, packed, stems removed

- A cup of cubed ice

- A scoop neutral flavored protein powder

- A teaspoon of Maca powder

- A cup of almond milk

i. Combine all the ingredients in a blender

ii. Blend thoroughly until smooth.

Vegan Butter Coffee

- A cup high quality brewed coffee

- A tablespoon of coconut butter

- A tablespoon of plant-based milk of your choice

Optional add-ins:

- 1 teaspoon of MCT oil

- 1 teaspoon of cinnamon

- 1 teaspoon of vanilla powder

- 1 teaspoon of coconut milk powder (instead of the plant milk)

Instructions

i. Brew your coffee – either a French press or automatic coffee maker using high-quality coffee.

ii. Add a cup of coffee in a blender along with coconut butter and other add-ins and blend until foamy.

iii. Pour in a mug and top with foamed plant milk or dust with cinnamon.

Lemon Lime Lavender Smoothie

- 1½ cups of plant yogurt

- 3 tablespoons of lemon juice

- 4 tablespoons of lime juice

- A drop of lavender extract, culinary OR ½ teaspoon of culinary lavender buds¼ cup of ice cubes

- ½ teaspoon of turmeric (or more to achieve desired color)

- ¼ cup of shavings from fresh organic lemons and limes

Instructions

i. Combine all the ingredients in a blender and serve chilled with citrus shavings and lavender buds on top for a strong scent as you spoon!

ii. Add some plant-based milk to thin mixture.

Cinnamon Apple Smoothie

Ingredients

- 1 small apple, sliced

- ½ cup of rolled oats

- ½ teaspoon of cinnamon

- ½ teaspoon of nutmeg

- 1 tablespoon almond butter

- ½ cup of unsweetened coconut milk

- 3 to 4 ice cubes

- ½ cup of cold water

Instructions

i. Combine oats and water in a blender and let it rest for a couple of minutes so the oats can soften.

ii. Add all the remaining ingredients to the blender and process for about 30 seconds until smooth.

iii. Pour into a glass and sprinkle with a little extra cinnamon and nutmeg. Enjoy!

iii.

Jalapeno Lime and Mango Protein Smoothie

- A small banana

- 1 Cheri-bundi Tart Cherry Mango smoothie pack (or ¾ cup frozen mango)

- A heaping tablespoon of chopped jalapeño (about ½ a small pepper)

- 1 cup unsweetened original almond milk (or coconut milk)

- 1 tablespoon flaxseed, ground

- 1 tablespoon chia seeds, ground

- 2 tablespoons hemp seed, ground

- ½ lime, freshly squeezed

- ½ an avocado (optional)

i. Combine all the ingredients in a blender and process for about 45 seconds until smooth.

ii. Pour into a glass and enjoy!

Apple Spinach Protein Smoothie

Ingredients

- 1 large organic apple

- 3 to 4 cups of organic spinach

- A tablespoon of organic almond butter

- 1 scoop (or packet) Vega Sport vanilla protein powder

- 1 cup of unsweetened original almond milk

- 4 to 5 ice cubes

Instructions

i. Add all the ingredients except spinach to a blender and process until smooth.

ii. Add spinach in batches, blending a handful at a time until it is all incorporated.

iii. Pour into a glass and enjoy!

Chapter 8: Snacks and Salads Recipes

Herbed Hummus

Ingredients

- A cup of fresh basil leaves, lightly packed and blanched

- ½ cup of fresh tarragon leaves, lightly packed and blanched

- 4 cups of cooked garbanzo beans

- 1 cup of vegetable broth

- ½ cup fresh flat-leaf parsley leaves, lightly packed

- Juice of 1 lemon

- 2 tablespoons of sesame seeds, toasted

- 2 cloves garlic

- ¼ cup of chopped chives

Instructions

i. Pat the basil and tarragon dry and coarsely chop them and combine in a blender.

ii. Add in beans, broth, parsley, lemon juice, sesame seeds, and garlic and continue processing until the desired consistency is achieved.

iii. Stir in the chives. Enjoy. This can be stored for up to 4 days.

Herby Crust Asparagus Spears

Ingredients

- 1 bunch of asparagus

- 2 tablespoons of hemp seeds

- ¼ cup of nutritional yeast

- 1 teaspoon of garlic powder or 3 garlic cloves, minced

- 1/8 teaspoon of ground pepper

- Pinch of paprika

- ¼ cup of whole wheat breadcrumbs

- Juice of ½ a lemon

Instructions

i. Preheat the oven to 350°F.

ii. Wash the asparagus and remove the white bottom end.

iii. Transfer hemp seeds to a small bowl and mix in the nutritional yeast, garlic, pepper, paprika, and breadcrumbs. Stir and set aside.

iv. In a baking dish, place the asparagus spears side by side sprinkle over hemp mixture.

v. Bake for 20 to 30 minutes to achieve crispy asparagus.

vi. Serve and sprinkle with some lemon juice.

Green Pea Guacamole

- 2 cups of frozen green peas, thawed

- 1 teaspoon crushed garlic

- ¼ cup of fresh lime juice

- ½ teaspoon of ground cumin

- 1 tomato, chopped

- 4 green onions, chopped

- ½ cup of chopped fresh cilantro

- ⅛ of a teaspoon of hot sauce

- Sea salt to taste

i. Blend the peas, garlic, lime juice, and cumin in a food processor until smooth.

ii. Stir in the tomato, green onion, cilantro, and hot sauce and transfer into a bowl. Season as desired.

iii. Cover and refrigerate for half an hour before serving.

Summer Chickpea Salad

- 2 to 2½ tablespoons of freshly squeezed lemon juice

- 1 tablespoons of pure maple syrup

- 1 teaspoon of Dijon mustard

- ½ teaspoon of salt

- ½ teaspoon of lemon zest, optional

- 2 cups cooked chickpeas

- 1 cup tomatoes cut in bite-size chunks

- 1 cup avocado cut in bite-sized chunks

- ½ cup Kalamata olives sliced

- 1½ to 2 cups of fresh spinach leaves roughly chopped

- ¼ cup torn/chopped basil leaves

- 1 to 2 tablespoons of chopped chives, optional

Instructions

i. In a large bowl, whisk together the lemon juice; a few drops at a time; with maple syrup, Dijon, salt, and lemon zest.

ii. Add the chickpeas, tomatoes, avocado, olives, spinach, basil and chives.

iii. Toss the mixture gently to prevent the avocado from mushing up. Add lemon juice to achieve the desired tang.

iv. Season as desired with salt or pepper and serve

Jicama and Spinach Salad Recipe

Ingredients

For Salad:

- 10 ounces baby spinach, washed and dried

- 1 jicama, washed, peeled and cut in strips

- 16 grape or cherry tomatoes, cut in half

- 12 green or Kalamata olives, chopped

- 4 teaspoons raw or roasted sunflower seeds

- 8 teaspoons walnuts, chopped

- Maple Mustard Dressing

For Dressing:

- 4 heaping tablespoons Dijon mustard

- 2 tablespoon maple syrup (plus more to taste, if desired)

- 2 cloves garlic, minced

- 1 to 2 tablespoons water

- ¼ teaspoon sea salt

- Dash cayenne pepper

i. For salad, top spinach with jicama, tomatoes and chopped olives. Sprinkle with some sunflower seeds and walnuts as desired.

ii. For the dressing: Whisk all ingredients together in small mixing bowl until emulsified. Taste and add more maple syrup if sweeter dressing is desired.

iii. Drizzle the dressing over each salad. Serve immediately.

Mint Chip Energy Bites

- 1/8 teaspoon peppermint extract

- Pinch of fine sea salt

- 2 tablespoons mini chocolate chips

- 10 Medjool dates, pitted

- ½ cup of coconut flakes

- ½ cup of chopped walnuts

- ¼ cup of cocoa powder

Instructions

i.   Add dates to your food processor and process until broken up into pea-sized bits.

ii. Add in coconut flakes, walnuts, cocoa powder, peppermint extract, and a pinch of salt and continue processing until it is well-combined into a large ball.

iii. Roll the mixture into roughly 1-inch balls and freeze for 20 minutes then transfer to refrigerator.

No-Bake Brownie Energy Bites

Ingredients

Dry Ingredients:

- ½ cup gluten-free oat flour

- ½ cup unsweetened cocoa powder

- ¼ cup ground flaxseed

- ½ cup vegan chocolate chips

Wet Ingredients:

- ¾ cup natural, unsalted creamy almond butter

- ¼ cup pure maple syrup

- 1 teaspoon pure vanilla extract

Instructions

i.   In a large bowl, mix together all of the dry ingredients: oat flour, cocoa powder, flaxseed and chocolate chips.

ii. Add vanilla, maple syrup and almond butter whilst stirring and folding using a spatula.

iii. Using a cookie scoop, scoop and drop a ball into your hands. Roll and press into bites. Enjoy!

Dairy-Free Banana Nut Muffins

Ingredients

Dry Ingredients:

- 1½ cups of gluten-free oat flour

- ¾ cup of almond meal

- ¾ teaspoon of baking powder

- ½ teaspoon of baking soda

- ¼ teaspoon of salt

Wet Ingredients:

- 3 medium, very ripe bananas (1 cup mashed)

- ¼ cup of melted coconut oil

- ¼ cup of coconut sugar

- 1 flax egg (1 tablespoon ground flax + 3 tablespoons water, whisk together, set for 15 mins)

- 1 teaspoon of pure vanilla extract

Add-ins:

- ¾ cup walnuts, chopped

- Optional for topping

- 2 tablespoons walnuts, chopped

Instructions

i. Preheat the oven to 350°F and line a 12-cup muffin pan with muffin liners.

ii. Add peeled bananas to a bowl and mash until they are smooth. Whisk in the flax egg, coconut oil, coconut sugar, and vanilla.

iii. Continue whisking in oat flour, almond meal, baking powder, baking soda and salt until well-incorporated then fold in walnuts.

iv. Using a large scoop, scoop and drop batter evenly into muffin cups.

v. Bake for about 20 minutes and set aside to cool on a cooling rack.

No-Bake Sweet Potato Chocolate Chip Cookies

Ingredients

- A cup of dates pitted and softened

- ½ cup of creamy almond or cashew butter

- ½ cup of cooked and mashed or pureed sweet potato

- 1 teaspoon of pure vanilla extract

- ¼ teaspoon of cinnamon

- A pinch salt

- 7 to 8 tablespoons of organic coconut flour

- 1/3 cup of mini chocolate chips

Instructions

i. Add your dates to the bowl of a food processor and process on high until a paste forms.

ii. Once you achieve the pasty consistency, add the mashed sweet potato, nut butter, vanilla, cinnamon and process until blended.

iii. Stir in 7 tablespoons of the coconut flour until a thick dough forms, then chill the dough in the freezer for 20 minutes

iv. If the dough is still very sticky, stir in some more of the coconut flour.

v. Fold in the mini chocolate chips, and then roll the dough into balls or cookie shapes. They will have a cookie dough-like texture and are best stored in the refrigerator. Enjoy!

Potato Pancakes

- 2 russet potatoes, grated

- 1 large zucchini, grated

- ½ yellow onion, grated

- ½ cup of oat flour

- A teaspoon of baking powder

- ½ teaspoon of freshly ground black pepper

i. Preheat oven to 420 degrees. Cover two sheet pans with parchment paper.

ii. Spread half of the grated vegetables on a clean kitchen towel, then roll and wring the towel to draw out the excess moisture.

iii. Transfer to a large mixing bowl. Repeat with the remaining vegetables.

iv. In a small bowl, combine the oat flour, baking powder, and pepper and add to the vegetable bowl, and mix well, using your hands to evenly distribute the flour and baking powder.

v. Scoop some of the potato mixture, and hand-shape it into a semi-tight ball. Flatten with your palms, and place the pancake onto the prepared pan. Repeat with the remaining mix, spacing the pancakes appropriately.

vi. Bake for no more than 15 minutes. Flip and bake for another 10 or so minutes. Top with the condiment of your choice.

BONUS: Make Your Plant-Based Lifestyle a Success

Key Pillars Going Forward

Water

Water contains no calories, fat, or cholesterol and is low in sodium. It is nature's appetite suppressant, and it helps the body to metabolize fat thereby helping you lose weight.

Fiber

There are a slew of health benefits that come with consuming lots of dietary fiber. They include:

 Normalizing bowel movements and maintaining bowel health

 Lower blood cholesterol levels

 Helps control blood sugar levels

 Promote healthier gut bacteria

Reduce risk of certain cancers

Rest and Sleep

Going forward, adequate rest and sleep will become a major pillar in your quest to lead a healthy lifestyle. The importance of sleep and rest cannot be overstated. Among its numerous benefits include:

 Appetite regulation

 Reducing your calorie intake

 Increases your resting metabolism

 Prevents insulin resistance

 Provide you with energy for physical activity

Positive Mindset

A positive mindset can help you maintain your plant-based diet and realize your health and fitness goals. Seeing as this requires patience and commitment, having a positive outlook and approach is going to help you: stay motivated, focus on the positive aspects of your diet and overcome emotions during your low moments.

Physical Activity

The health benefits of regular exercise and physical activity are hard to ignore. Exercising regularly will help you:

▢ Control weight

▢ Fight off health conditions and diseases

▢ Improve your mood

▢ Boost your energy levels

▢ Promote better sleep

Tips for Lazy Days and Dining Out

We all know that eating out can sometimes be challenging when you are following a whole food, plant-based diet and avoiding oil and other concentrated ingredients or if you need to eat gluten-free. On the other hand, ordering takeout or dine-in can be quite convenient after a long, hectic day where prepping food was simply not in your plans. So, here are some tips you can use when dining out.

    i.   Look up niche restaurants such as plant-based restaurants or vegan restaurants

    ii.   Specify how you want your meals prepared. Always opt for steamed, baked, water sautéed or grilled

    iii. Play nice with the wait staff to get them to make your preferences happen.

Conclusion

I believe now you understand how a plant-based diet lifestyle can be beneficial to you. I hope that the book answered all questions you may have heard about this style of dieting and that you can start to make it work for you. If you are still hesitant about entirely giving up animal products, you don't have to. The main take away here is that you make plant-based meals the main part of your diet as you make baby steps to transition into a full plant-based lifestyle. You will soon realize that your body and mind start to feel better, stronger and healthier. You can't fix your health until you fix your diet!

CPSIA information can be obtained
at www.ICGtesting.com
Printed in the USA
LVHW100036291220
675246LV00006B/107